# O A P N

OXFORD AMERICAN POCKET NOTES

# Diagnosis and Treatment of Overactive Bladder

# O A P N

OXFORD AMERICAN POCKET NOTES

# Diagnosis and Treatment of Overactive Bladder

By

**Jerry G. Blaivas, MD**
Clinical Professor of Urology
Weill Cornell Medical School
Adjunct Professor of Urology
SUNY – Downstate Medical School
New York, New York

**Rajveer Singh Purohit, MD, MPH**
Clinical Assistant Professor
Department of Urology
Weill Medical College of Cornell University
New York, New York

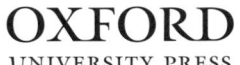

OXFORD
UNIVERSITY PRESS

# OXFORD
## UNIVERSITY PRESS

Oxford University Press, Inc., publishes works that further
Oxford University's objective of excellence
in research, scholarship, and education.

Oxford  New York

Auckland  Cape Town  Dar es Salaam  Hong Kong  Karachi
Kuala Lumpur  Madrid  Melbourne  Mexico City  Nairobi
New Delhi  Shanghai  Taipei  Toronto

With offices in

Argentina  Austria  Brazil  Chile  Czech Republic  France  Greece
Guatemala  Hungary  Italy  Japan Poland Portugal  Singapore
South Korea  Switzerland  Thailand  Turkey Ukraine  Vietnam

Copyright © 2011 by Oxford University Press, Inc.

Published by Oxford University Press, Inc.
198 Madison Avenue, New York, New York 10016
www.oup.com

ISBN: 978-0-19-975372-7

9  8  7  6  5  4  3  2  1
Printed in China
on acid-free paper

## DISCLOSURES

Dr. Blaivas is a stock holder of HDH and Endogun. He is also a consultant to Pfizer, Astellas, and Novasys.

## TABLE OF CONTENTS

## INTRODUCTION

The term *overactive bladder* (OAB) was first coined in the 1990s, to describe a constellation of lower urinary tract symptoms (LUTS) comprised of urinary frequency, urgency, urge incontinence, and nocturia. Overactive bladder is very common, and has a major negative impact on quality of life.[1,2] Because treatment had been notoriously ineffective in past decades, many patients "suffered in silence" and did not even seek medical care. There are a number of reasons for this. First, many patients were too embarrassed to discuss incontinence with their doctors. Second, the available treatments were largely ineffective. And, finally, because they had so little to offer, doctors were largely uninterested in treating these patients.

Fortunately, all this is changing. Increased advertising by the health care industry about OAB has resulted in widespread interest among physicians and patients alike. The resources to diagnose and treat OAB are expanding exponentially, and OAB treatment—once the province of the specialist—is increasingly in the hands of primary care providers (PCPs): over half of the prescriptions written for OAB drugs are written in the primary care setting. It is the purpose of this monograph to provide PCPs and other providers with the knowledge base and understanding of not only how to diagnose and treat OAB, but also when to refer to the specialist.

## INCIDENCE AND PREVALENCE

Several large epidemiological studies have reported a prevalence of OAB of 16%–17% in both the United States and

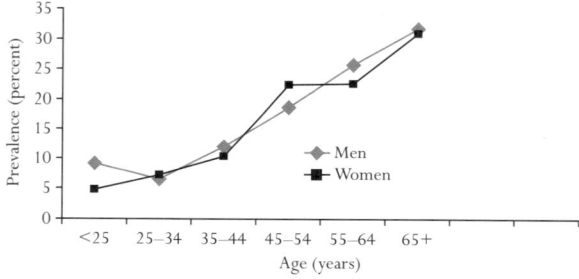

**Figure 1** Prevalence of overactive bladder (OAB) by age
From Stewart, W., et al. The prevalence and impact of overactive
bladder in the U.S: results from the NOBLE program. *Neurorol
Urodynam* 2001;20(406):8.

Europe.[1,2] The NOBLE study[2] was comprised of 17,231
random cold-call telephone interviews conducted in the
United States. Of these, 5,204 households completed the
telephone interview. The OAB prevalence was found to be
17%, of whom 37% had incontinence and 63% did not.
They also noted that the prevalence increases with age
(Figure 1).

## DEFINITION OF OVERACTIVE BLADDER

Overactive bladder is defined by The Standardization
Committee of International Continence Society (ICS)[3] as
"(urinary) urgency, with or without urge incontinence, usually with frequency and nocturia, can be described as the
overactive bladder syndrome.... These symptom com-
binations are suggestive of urodynamically demonstrable

detrusor overactivity, but can be due to other forms of ure-thro-vesical dysfunction."

Further, the committee recommended that the term OAB should be used only "if there is no proven infection or other obvious pathology."

They go on to describe urgency as "the complaint of a sudden compelling desire to pass urine, which is difficult to defer." However, these definitions may be too restrictive for clinical utility. Accordingly, here, we propose broader definitions of urgency and OAB that we believe are more relevant.

When patients are specifically asked what they mean by urgency, many describe symptoms that do not conform to the ICS definition. In a study designed to define the sensation of urgency, patients were asked to describe, in their own words, what they meant by urgency.[4] The most common answer was, "If I wait too long, I have trouble getting to the bathroom in time." In fact, only a minority of patients described urgency as a "sudden" event. Based on these data, two distinct types of urgency emerged that may have relevance for the choice of treatment. Type 1 was described as an intensification of the normal urge to void, and occurred in 69% of patients with OAB. We refer to type 1 as *sensory urgency*. Type 2 was a sudden precipitous urge that is a different sensation from the normal urge, and which conformed to the ICS definition. Type 2 urgency occurred in 31%. We presume that type 2 urgency is caused by detrusor overactivity (an involuntary bladder contraction). Based on these data, we propose a modified definition of urgency: *A compelling sensation of the need to pass urine, which is difficult to defer.*

The ICS definition considers OAB to be a syndrome, with symptoms suggestive of detrusor overactivity (involuntary contractions of the bladder), and recommends that the term OAB be used only "if there is no proven infection or other obvious pathology." This definition may also be too restrictive—OAB should be considered a symptom complex, not a syndrome. A *syndrome* is a group of symptoms that together are characteristic of a specific disorder or disease, such as Down syndrome (trisomy 21); a *symptom complex* is a group of symptoms that commonly occur together but require evaluation to determine the diagnosis. The distinction between a symptom complex and a syndrome is more than mere semantics because, unless a remediable cause of a patient's symptom complex is sought, the patient will be treated empirically and denied the possibility of a "cure." That a differential diagnosis of OAB exists, and that remediable conditions cause the symptoms is unquestioned and is discussed later. For example, in men, the commonest cause of OAB is benign prostatic hypertrophy (BPH) and prostatic obstruction,[5] and surgical relief of the obstruction cures the OAB in over 50% of patients.[6,7] Further, detrusor overactivity is only demonstrable in 40%–60% of patients with OAB.[8,9] That means that, in many OAB patients, the symptoms might not be caused by involuntary detrusor contractions at all. Other possible causes include sensory abnormalities and bladder irritants that make it uncomfortable to delay micturition.

Our proposed clinical definition of OAB: *Overactive bladder is a symptom complex comprised of urinary urgency with or without other symptoms such as urinary frequency, nocturia, urge incontinence, and lower urinary tract pain.*

## CLINICAL PRESENTATIONS OF OVERACTIVE BLADDER

Overactive bladder presents in one of two ways: (1) The patient complains that "I have OAB," because he or she is familiar with the term from advertisements, the Internet, or other patients and doctors; or (2) The patient complains of symptoms that the physician interprets as OAB.

The cornerstone of OAB is *urinary urgency*, redefined as "a compelling sensation of the need to pass urine, which is difficult to defer." *Urge incontinence* is incontinence that is immediately preceded by urgency. *Urinary frequency* is simply defined as the need to urinate more often than normal. *Nocturia* is the complaint that the individual has to wake at night one or more times to void.

- *Urinary frequency.* Urinary frequency is defined as voiding more than eight times in 24 hours,[10,11] but there is great variability in both men and women depending largely on how much urine is excreted (see Table 1). In general, the greater the 24-hour urine output, the greater the number of voids. However, some patients with larger 24-hour volumes adapt to having larger volumes per void, so they void less frequently than would be expected.[12] For an individual patient, though, urinary frequency is voiding more often than he or she is comfortable with. For an accurate history of urinary frequency, a *bladder diary* is nearly indispensable and will be discussed in a later section.

**Table 1** Normal Urinary Outputs

| Variable | All Patients Mean (Median) | Male Mean (Median) | Female Mean (Median) |
|---|---|---|---|
| Volume Day mL* | | 1267 (1,105) | 1261 (721) |
| Volume Night mL* | | 446 (408) | 468 (414) |
| Frequency Day* | | 6.1 (6.0) | 6.7 (6.5) |
| Frequency Night* | | 0.4 (0.3) | 0.4 (0.3) |
| Bladder Capacity day* | | 250 (234) | 229 (220) |
| Bladder Capacity night* | | 334 (309) | 332 (294) |
| 24-hr Volume | 1,730 (1,576) | 1,713 (1,512) | 1,729 (1619) |
| 24-hr Frequency | 7.1 (7.0) | 6.5 (6.3) | 7.1 (6.8) |
| Bladder Capacity day† | 81 (75) | | 81 (47) |
| Bladder Capacity night† | 514 (480) | | 514 (190) |

Extrapolated from

* Amundsen, CL., et al. Bladder diary measurements in asymptomatic females: functional bladder capacity, frequency, and 24-hr volume. *Neurourol Urodyn* 2007; 26(3):341–9.

† Parsons, M., et al. Normative bladder diary measurements: night versus day. Bladder Diary Research Team. *Neurourol Urodyn* 2007;26(4):465–73.

- *Nocturia.* Simply put, nocturia is awakening during sleep hours to void. The prevalence of nocturia in adults ranges from 38% to 60% in men and 36% to 55% in women; 11%–28% experience two or more voids at night. Regardless of gender, ethnicity, and race, the prevalence of nocturia increases with age.[13–17]

- *Urinary urgency.* As defined earlier, urinary urgency is the sensation of the need to pass urine, which is difficult to defer. The intensity of the sensation of the need to void is variable and can be graded. There are several validated methods of grading urgency[18–20]; we recommend the Urge Perception Score (UPS) depicted in Table 2.[18]

**Table 2** Urge Perception Score

- **Type 0 - No urge**
- **Type 1 - Mild urge (can delay for >1 hour)**
- **Type 2 - Moderate urge (can delay for 10–60 minutes)**
- **Type 3 - Severe urge (can delay for <10 minutes)**
- **Type 4 - Precipitous urge (must void immediately)**

From Blaivas, J.G., et al. The urgency perception score: validation and test-retest. *J Urol*, 2007;177(1):199–202.

The UPS can be used to grade individual micturitions in a bladder diary or as a general descriptor to describe the severity of the patient's urge symptom.

- *Urge incontinence.* Urge incontinence is a urine loss that is associated with the sensation of urgency.
- *"Door key" or "garage door syndrome."* Urinary urgency and/ or urge incontinence can be triggered by certain conditions, in what appears to be a conditioned reflex. The most dramatic example of this is the "door key" or "garage door syndrome," which is characterized by UPS grade 3–4 urgency that occurs when the patient's car pulls into the driveway or when putting the key into the front door lock. A more common scenario is the urge to void that many people experience when they are close to or hear the sound of running water.

## DIFFERENTIAL DIAGNOSIS OF OVERACTIVE BLADDER

In both sexes, urinary tract infection is the commonest cause of OAB symptoms. A fairly complete list of the differential diagnosis is depicted in Table 3, but it is somewhat different in men and women. In a study of 122 consecutive men

**Table 3** Differential Diagnosis of Overactive Bladder (OAB)

**Non-neurogenic**

Cystitis – bacterial, fungal, tuberculous, bilharzial, radiation, idiopathic
Bladder outlet obstruction
   Men – bladder neck*, prostate*, urethral stricture*
   Women – pelvic organ prolapse*, postsurgical*, bladder neck*, stricture*
Stress incontinence* (women)
Pelvic organ prolapse* (women)
Bladder cancer*
Bladder stones*
Bladder foreign body* (postsurgical erosion of slings and sutures)

**Neurogenic**

Supraspinal neurological lesions
   Stroke
   Parkinson disease
   Hydrocephalus*
   Brain tumor
   Traumatic brain injury
   Multiple sclerosis
Suprasacral spinal lesions
   Herniated disc*
   Spinal cord injury
   Spinal cord tumor
   Multiple sclerosis
   Myelodysplasia
   Transverse myelitis

**Idiopathic**

The diagnoses marked by * are potentially reversible by surgical intervention.

with OAB, the two commonest causes were BPH (32%) and bladder outlet obstruction (22%)[21]; in fact, truly idiopathic OAB was found in only 5% of this population. Many other studies have documented this differential diagnosis in men, including bladder tumor, postsurgical pathology, and bladder stones.[5,22–24] Neurogenic etiologies of OAB include cerebrovascular accident, Parkinson disease, multiple sclerosis, spinal cord injury, and myelodysplasia.[25–27]

In women, the commonest cause of OAB after urinary tract infection is pelvic organ prolapse (POP). Sphincteric (stress) incontinence is very common in patients with OAB, and successful treatment of stress incontinence ameliorates the OAB symptoms in about 80%.[28] Other important causes include urethral obstruction and bladder cancer (see Table 3).

Another way of looking at the differential diagnosis is to consider the causes of the individual symptoms of OAB.

### Urinary Frequency
The frequency of urination depends on three basic factors: the 24-hour urinary output, the bladder capacity, and psychosocial considerations.

### Volume of Urinary Output
Table 1 depicts normal values for urinary output, which is highly variable and depends almost entirely on intake of fluid and food (most foods are 60%–90% water). Urinary output is regulated by metabolic needs and pathologic conditions. Normally, urine excretion is about 70% of oral fluid intake,[29] but output can be greatly diminished by abnormal fluid losses due to excessive sweating (from exercise, exposure to high temperature, tachypnea, etc.). Edema is also, in a sense, an abnormal fluid loss from the intravascular space. Diuretic use and liquids that contain diuretics (such as caffeine) increase urine output.

### Bladder Capacity

Bladder capacity is the maximum urine volume that a patient can comfortably hold. Bladder capacity can be assessed by two different techniques: the bladder diary and cystometry.

The bladder diary is recorded by the patient and includes the time and volume of each urination over a specified period of time, usually 1 day.[30] The patient is given a preprinted diary form to fill out contemporaneously and is asked to void each time into a measuring cup. The maximum voided volume (MVV) is the largest voided volume reported in the diary. Normal values for MVV are seen in Table 1.

*Cystometric bladder capacity* (CBC) is the volume at which the patient feels he or she can no longer delay micturition during cystometry. The CBC depends on a number of technical factors and may be at great variance from the MVV.[31, 32] It is mostly of interest to specialists.

In a series of diaries from 300 normal people, the median MVV was 330 mL (mean 204 mL), and the range of capacities was large (90–1,020 mL), with the 95th percentile of MVV at 679 mL (see Table 1).[11] Some people, though, do not completely empty their bladders, so the actual bladder capacity is the MVV + post-void residual urine volume (PVR). For most patients, PVR is clinically irrelevant, but it should be part of the basic evaluation because it may be the only sign of severe urethral obstruction or impaired detrusor contractility—two conditions that demand specific treatment and careful follow-up.

Theoretically, a patient need not void any more often than his 24-hour voided volume divided by MVV, but in fact that is rarely the case. Most people only attain their MVV once or twice a day, usually during sleep. The rest of the time, they void because factors other than bladder volume trigger the sensation of the need to void. For example, in some people, spicy foods or caffeine (independent of the diuretic effect) causes a strong urge to void at low bladder volumes. Psychosocial and environmental factors, such as being distracted by activities (exercise, intense concentration) can increase the bladder volume at which the urge to void is perceived. Finally, a large number of pathologic conditions, such as urinary tract infection and urethral obstruction, can affect bladder capacity.

### Psychosocial Factors

Psychosocial factors also play a major role in the frequency of urination. There is a popular perception that constant water intake is healthy. Some people drink excessive amounts of water to aid in dieting, to prevent kidney stones, and some may suffer from psychogenic polydipsia. Unless there is a specific medical reason to do so, patients with urinary frequency who drink excessive amounts should be advised to cut back and drink according to thirst.

### Nocturia

The etiology of nocturia is divided into four broad categories defined by calculations made from the bladder diary[33–35]: (1) nocturnal polyuria (NP), (2) low nocturnal bladder capacity (NBC), (3) mixed (a combination of NP and low bladder capacity), and (4) global polyuria (Table 4).

**Table 4** Differential Diagnosis in Women (Excluding Bacterial Cystitis)

| Diagnosis* | Number (%) |
|---|---|
| Mixed stress and urge incontinence | 38 (32%) |
| Pelvic organ prolapse | 28 (23%) |
| Idiopathic | 21 (17%) |
| Urinary tract infection | 19 (16%) |
| Neurogenic | 16 (13%) |
| Miscellaneous | 11 (9%) |
| Prior pelvic surgery | 36 (30%) |
| Urethral obstruction | 22 (18%) |

* Adds up to more than 100% because some patients had more than one diagnosis.

To understand the differential diagnosis, some terms need to be defined. *Nocturnal urine volume* (NUV) is the volume of urine voided throughout the night including the first morning void. However, the first morning void is considered a daytime void and is not included with the tally of nightly voids. The *nocturia index* (Ni) is calculated by dividing NUV by MVV.[34,35] When the Ni is >1, NUV exceeds bladder capacity, and nocturia or enuresis occurs.[34,35] An increased Ni may be due to either NP, low nocturnal bladder capacity, or both. The nocturnal polyuria *index* (NPi) is defined as NUV divided by the 24-hour urine volume; that is, it is the percentage of urine produced during sleep hours.

*Global polyuria*, which may cause both day- and nighttime urinary frequency, is defined as a 24-hour urine output of >40 mL/kg body weight. Global polyuria may be due to pathologic causes, such as diabetes mellitus, diabetes insipidus, or polydipsia, or it may be due to psychosocial or behavioral aberrations, as discussed earlier.

*Nocturnal polyuria* is increased production of urine at night.[33–37] Normally, there is an age-dependent circadian pattern of urine production. The mean NPi is 0.14 in people <25 years of age, and this rises to 0.34 in those >65 years of age.[38] Other criteria for nocturnal polyuria include an NUV of >6.4 mL/kg and nocturnal urine output of >0.9 mL/min.[39] There are numerous causes of nocturnal polyuria, including excessive evening fluid intake, peripheral edema, congestive heart failure, diabetes mellitus, and obstructive sleep apnea.[15,17,33–35,37–47] A complete list is seen in Table 6.

*Decreased nocturnal bladder capacity* may be associated with a global decrease in MVV or a bladder capacity that is reduced only at night. In both conditions, the nighttime urinary volume exceeds bladder capacity, and the patient is awakened by the need to void because the bladder does not hold enough. Causes of both types are the same as those for OAB (see Table 3).

*Mixed nocturia*, which affects many patients with nocturia, is a combination of NP and low NBC. In a study of 194 patients, nocturia was due to NP in 7%, low NBC in 57%, global polyuria in 23%, and a mixture of NP and low NBC in 36%.[35]

### Urgency and Urge Incontinence
The differential diagnosis of urgency and urge incontinence is the same as that for OAB and is depicted in Tables 5 and 6.

**Table 5** Differential Diagnosis in Men

| Differential Diagnosis | Number (%) |
| --- | --- |
| BPH | 40 (32) |
| BPO | 27 (22) |
| Prostate cancer complications | 25 (20) |
| Neurogenic bladder | 13 (11) |
| Urethral stricture | 7 (06) |
| Idiopathic OAB | 6 (05) |
| Bladder stone | 2 (02) |
| Bladder cancer | 1 (01) |
| Bladder diverticulum | 1 (01) |
| Total | 122 (100) |

**Table 6** Etiology of Nocturia

| Classification of Nocturia | Etiology |
| --- | --- |
| Nocturnal polyuria | Congestive heart failure<br>Diabetes mellitus<br>Obstructive sleep apnea<br>Peripheral edema/venous stasis<br>Nephrotic syndrome/Hypoalbuminemia<br>Hepatic failure<br>Excessive nighttime fluid intake |
| Diminished NBC | Prostatic obstruction<br>Nocturnal detrusor overactivity<br>Neurogenic bladder<br>Cancer of bladder, prostate, or urethra<br>Acquired voiding dysfunction/Anxiety disorders<br>Pharmacologic agents (eg cholinergic agonists)<br>Bladder & ureteral stones |
| Global Polyuria | Diabetes mellitus & insipidus<br>Primary or acquired polydipsia |

## DIAGNOSTIC EVALUATION

Clinicians treat individual patients, one at a time, not populations of patients. When it comes to treating the individual patient, the more the physician knows about him or her, the more accurate the diagnosis and the more effective the treatment. As a general rule, knowing more costs more—both in time and money—and most health care workers do not have access to enough of either to know as much about a patient as they would like. The result is that, in most patients with OAB, initial treatment is empiric, often based on diagnostic and treatment algorithms.

The following sections provide a diagnostic and treatment algorithm that highlights the role of the PCP. The goals of the workup are to ensure that the patient actually has OAB and to exclude important and/or remediable conditions, such as urinary retention and bladder cancer, which require urgent treatment.

### History

The history begins with a detailed account of the precise nature of the patient's urinary symptoms. Questionnaires, bladder diaries, and pad tests for incontinence are very useful adjuncts and are best utilized prior to history taking. The examiner should not rely on any one of these tools, but rather, use each as confirmation of the other.

The patient should be asked how often he urinates during the day and night, and how long micturition can be postponed once he gets the urge. Why does he void as often as he does? Is it because of severe urge, or out of convenience, or as an attempt to prevent incontinence? Is there urgency or urge incontinence? Stress incontinence? If so, is urine lost only for an instant during the stress, or is there uncontrollable voiding? Are protective pads worn? Do they become saturated? How often are they changed? Is there difficulty initiating the stream, requiring pushing or straining to start? Is the stream weak or interrupted? Has the patient ever been in urinary retention?

In women, POP may present with a spectrum of LUTS ranging from urinary retention to OAB to stress incontinence. The patient may feel or see a protrusion from the vagina or feel like she is "sitting on a ball." There may be a pressure sensation in the vagina, rectum, or groin. There may be a sacral backache that resolves when the patient is lying down.[48] Many patients, though, even with severe prolapse, are not aware of it at all and simply present with OAB symptoms or other LUTS.

## Past Medical History

The patient should be specifically queried about neurologic conditions such as multiple sclerosis, spinal cord injury, lumbar disc disease, myelodysplasia, diabetes, stroke, and Parkinson disease. If there is not a previously diagnosed neurologic disease, it is important to ask about double vision, muscular weakness, paralysis or poor coordination, tremor, numbness, and tingling. A history of prostate or vaginal surgery should suggest the possibility of urethral obstruction or erosion of mesh into the urinary tract. Radiation therapy may cause a small-capacity, low-compliance bladder, or radiation cystitis.

### Bladder Questionnaire

Questionnaires expedite the retrieval of all of this information but do not supplant the medical history. Each should supplement the other, and final judgment about the nature of symptoms should be attained by resolving conflicts between questionnaire, bladder diary, pad tests, and anamnestic responses. Two questionnaires are helpful in the clinical setting. One is directed toward a general medical overview, and the second includes a detailed account of urinary symptoms. Patients are encouraged to complete these questionnaires prior to the office visit, thus offering them the opportunity to ponder the questions and to acquire information, such as the names of medications and dates of previous surgeries, prior to the office visit. One such questionnaire is the Overactive Bladder Symptom Score,[49] which is depicted in Appendix A.

### Bladder Diary

To document the nature and severity of urinary symptoms, a bladder diary is indispensable.[10,30,50,51] The particular information recorded in the diary depends on the patient's symptoms, but all diaries should include at least the time and amount of each micturition. From such a diary, the following information can be calculated: (1) the total, day- and nighttime urinary output; (2) the number of day- and nighttime voids; and (3) the largest and lowest voided volume. In addition, notations about the characterization, time, and severity of incontinence; the need to push or strain to void; and associated pain or urgency can be compiled.

An example of an OAB diary can be found in Appendix B.

## Pad Tests

A number of pad tests have been described, [30, 52] but for routine clinical purposes a simple 24-hour test during which the patient wears pads, changes them at will, and puts all of them into a plastic bag, is recommended. Observation alone is sufficient for routine purposes; for more sophisticated evaluation, the weight of an unused pad is multiplied by the number of pads changed and subtracted from the combined weight of all the wet pads. A weight of <8 g/24 hours is normal (due to sweat, secretions, etc.). [30, 53]

## Physical Examination

The physical examination begins by observing the patient's gait and demeanor as he or she first enters the office. A slight limp or lack of coordination, an abnormal speech pattern, facial asymmetry, or other abnormalities may be subtle signs of a neurologic condition. The abdomen should be examined for masses and a distended bladder. A pelvic examination is performed with the bladder comfortably full in lithotomy position. The patient is asked to cough or strain to reproduce symptoms of incontinence and to assess for POP. Grade 3 and 4 prolapse[54] is a potentially remediable cause of OAB.[30] The sacral dermatomes are evaluated by assessing anal sphincter tone and control, perianal sensation, and the bulbocavernosus reflex. With a finger in the rectum, the patient is asked to squeeze as if he or she was in the middle of urinating and trying to stop. A lax or weakened anal sphincter or the inability to voluntarily contract and relax are signs of neurologic damage. The bulbocavernosus reflex is checked by suddenly squeezing the glans penis or clitoris and feeling (or seeing) the anal sphincter and perineal muscles contract. The absence of this reflex in men is almost always associated with a neurologic lesion, but the reflex is not detectable in up to 30% of otherwise normal women.[55]

### Routine Laboratory Assessment

Routine laboratory studies begins with a urine dip stick. If pyuria or hematuria is indicated, a complete urinalysis, culture, and sensitivities should be ordered. Glycosuria suggests the possibility of diabetes mellitus that might be contributing to OAB symptoms. Positive urine cultures should be treated with culture-specific antibiotics, but patients with persistent bacteriuria or recurrent infections may require invasive testing while on antibiotics. Hematuria should be evaluated by upper-tract imaging (computed tomography [CT] scan of the abdomen and pelvis with and without IV contrast and a cystourethroscopy).

### Urodynamic Study

The main purpose of urodynamic investigation is to determine the pathophysiology underlying the patient's symptoms. Urodynamic technique varies from "eyeball urodynamics" to sophisticated multichannel synchronous video, pressure, and flow electromyography (EMG) studies. Synchronous multichannel video-urodynamics offer the most comprehensive, artifact-free means of arriving at a precise diagnosis,[5,56] but it is beyond the scope of this monograph.

### Eyeball Urodynamics

"Eyeball urodynamics" (Figure 2) is a simple method of assessing the cause of OAB in women that is performed

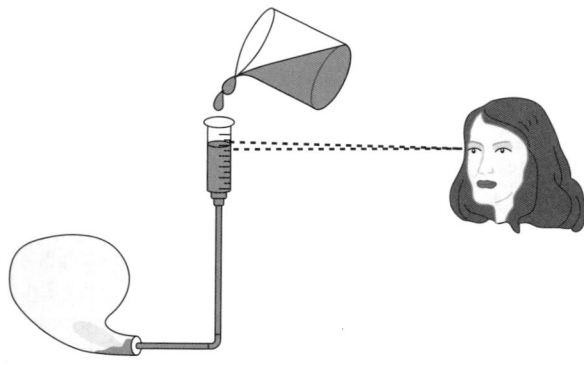

**Figure 2** Eyeball urodynamics.

in the office with only a catheter, a 60 mL syringe, and a bottle of sterile water or saline. The procedure is not recommended in men because urethral obstruction is very common and cannot be assessed with this technique. It is performed with the patient in the lithotomy position. The examiner should know the patient's history and the results of the bladder diary. The patient should be asked to void, a Foley catheter is inserted, and PVR is measured. A fluid reservoir (60 mL syringe with the barrel removed or irrigation bag) is connected and water or saline is then infused into the bladder by gravity. The reservoir is lowered and the meniscus observed at the height at which fluid inflow stops. The height of the meniscus above the symphysis pubis in centimeters is the resting intravesical pressure. The bladder is filled, and the patient is told to report her sensations to the examiner. When she perceives the urge to void, she is asked if that is the usual feeling that she experiences when she needs to urinate. Changes in intravesical pressure are apparent as a slowing down in the rate of fall, or a rise in the level of the fluid meniscus. A change in pressure may be caused by a detrusor contraction, an increase in abdominal pressure, or low bladder wall compliance. As soon as a change in pressure is noted, the examiner should attempt to determine the cause. Visual inspection will usually distinguish abdominal straining, but in doubtful cases the abdomen should be palpated. In most instances, the cause of the rise in intravesical pressure will be obvious, but when in doubt, formal cystometry with rectal pressure monitoring is necessary.

Any sudden rise in pressure that is accompanied by an urge to void or by incontinence is an involuntary detrusor contraction. In some instances, the etiology of the patient's incontinence is easily discernible as she voids uncontrollably around the catheter during an involuntary detrusor contraction. If involuntary detrusor contractions do not occur, the bladder is filled until the patient is comfortably full and the catheter is removed. The presence or absence of gravitational urinary loss is noted. The patient is asked to cough and bear down with gradually increasing force to determine the ease with which incontinence may be produced, and the vagina is inspected for signs of prolapse.

Incontinence that occurs during stress is not always due to sphincter abnormalities. In some patients, the stress initiates a reflex detrusor contraction. This condition has been termed *stress hyperreflexia*. Thus, it is important to determine whether the leakage occurs only during the stress and stops as soon as the stress is over, or if it continues uncontrollably. In the former case, the patient has stress incontinence; in the latter, it is stress hyperreflexia.

## TREATMENT

The most important aspects of treatment are to (1) attain an accurate diagnosis, (2) identify and treat remediable conditions, and (3) tailor the therapy to the underlying abnormality. With the exception of cystitis, the remediable conditions that cause OAB symptoms are beyond the purview of the nonspecialist. The treatment algorithm that we recommend is depicted in Figure 3.

### Cystitis

Cystitis means inflammation of the bladder. The most common cause of cystitis is infection with bacteria, but in rare cases, there may be infections due to tuberculosis, fungus, and other kinds of microorganisms. When bacterial infection is the cause, treatment with culture-specific antibiotics is usually curative within 48 hours. If symptoms persist longer than 5–7 days or recur shortly after successful treatment, there are a number of possibilities. First, the patient may not be taking the medicine properly. Second, the patient may have developed an infection with a resistant organism. Third, there may be other comorbidities, such as urethral obstruction, elevated PVR, urethral diverticulum, bladder cancer, bladder stones, or foreign body.

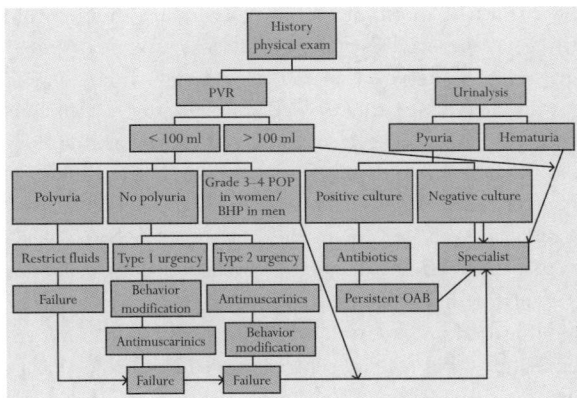

**Figure 3** Proposed treatment algorithm. POP = pelvic organ prolapse in women; BPH = signs and symptoms of prostatic obstruction in men; Type 1 urgency = a gradual onset of a compelling urge to void also known as sensory urgency; Type 2 urge = a sudden compelling urge to urinate, thought to be due to involuntary detrusor contractions.

Once bacterial infection has been excluded (or appropriately treated), if symptoms persist, the clinician needs to decide whether to treat the patient empirically, pursue further diagnostic evaluation as described earlier, or refer to a specialist.

### Empiric Treatments

For patients with new-onset OAB, empiric treatment is best accomplished after an OAB diary has been completed and overt remediable causes, such as urinary retention and high-grade prolapse, have been excluded. Even when a diary has not been done, treatment can be based on a clinical estimation of what the diary would look like.

Based on the diary and UPS, patients are divided into three presumptive groups: (1) sensory urgency (type 1 urgency), (2) detrusor overactivity (type 2 urgency), and (3) polyuria. For patients with polyuria, the treatment is straightforward: They are instructed to cut back on their oral intake of fluid (and high water-content foods like lettuce or fruit). If that fails to correct the polyuria, they should be evaluated for medical causes of polyuria, such as diabetes mellitus, diabetes insipidus, or polydipsia. For patients with presumed detrusor overactivity, behavior modification and/or anticholinergic medications are recommended. For patients with presumed idiopathic sensory urgency, behavior modification alone is recommended and if that fails, anticholinergic medication should be tried next.

### Behavior Modification

Behavior modification is an effective empiric therapy that deals with observable and measurable behaviors that cause and/or exacerbate symptoms and teaches the patient to change those behaviors. It consists of a number of techniques, including decreasing fluid intake, dietary and lifestyle changes, programmed voiding by the clock, and pelvic floor rehabilitation.[57] Behavioral therapies coupled with pharmacologic treatment have been shown to have a synergistic effect.[58]

We believe that behavioral therapies are effective in the great majority of patients who are motivated enough to pursue the program and can even be used when the symptoms are caused by diverse pathologic conditions, such as multiple sclerosis, prostatic obstruction, and Parkinson disease.

Regardless of the underlying cause, to the extent that the symptoms are related to bladder volume, decreasing fluid intake tends to improve OAB symptoms. Other behavioral modification principles are more complex and require a thorough evaluation of the bladder diary and urge perception scores for each void.

For patients with detrusor overactivity (DO), the goals are to teach how to prevent or abort the involuntary detrusor contractions. The first step is to determine whether the symptoms appear to be related to bladder volume; if they are, the patient is taught to void before the bladder reaches the critical volume that triggers detrusor overactivity. The second step is to teach the patient to recognize patterns that seem to cause the DO—running water, "key lock and garage door syndrome," etc. The third step is to teach the patient to contract his pelvic floor (Kegel maneuver) to prevent or abort involuntary detrusor contractions. Finally, the patient is taught to gradually increase the amount of urine that can be comfortably held in the bladder. This is a process that generally takes about 8–12 weeks and consists of diary keeping and the gradual and purposeful increase in intervoiding interval by about 15 minutes per week. Behavioral modification and bladder training have been shown to help over 50% of women who have incontinence secondary to detrusor instability and even in those with combination of detrusor instability and sphincteric incompetence.[59,60]

For patients with sensory urgency, the first step in the behavior modification process is to determine whether the symptom is related to bladder volume; if it is, the patient is taught to void before that critical volume is reached. The next step is to determine whether any dietary factors, such as caffeine, spicy foods, etc., provoke the symptoms and reduce or eliminate them from the diet. In some patients, psychosocial triggers such as stress or anxiety seem to exacerbate symptoms. The remainder of the program is the same as described for patients with DO.

## MEDICATIONS

Two basic classes of medications have been shown to be effective for the treatment of OAB symptoms: antimuscarinics and tricyclic antidepressants.

### Antimuscarinics

The mainstays of medical treatment for OAB are the antimuscarinic agents (AMA). Antimuscarinic agents block parasympathetic muscarinic receptors, of which there are five known subtypes: M1, M2, M3, M4, and M5. The rationale for choosing antimuscarinics for the treatment of OAB is based on the belief that involuntary detrusor contractions, also called detrusor overactivity (DO), are the root cause of OAB,[61] and that inhibition of DO is the goal of treatment—a hypothesis that recently has come under question, as described earlier. The M3 receptor, widely distributed throughout the bladder, is responsible for detrusor contraction.[62] M3 is also found in vascular and gut smooth muscle, the lungs, and in the iris, accounting for the common side effects of constipation and blurred vision.[63]

M2 has the highest receptor concentration in the bladder (and is also present in the heart), yet its role in bladder function is not well understood. Certain AMA's can prolong the QT interval, which has been associated with life-threatening ventricular tachycardia or torsades de pointes, and the resulting tachycardia can cause dizziness, syncope, cardiac arrest, and death.[64] This has been the most common cause of drug withdrawal over the last decade.[64] Other drugs that have been associated with QT prolongation include antibiotics (e.g., azithromycin), antifungals (e.g., ketoconazole), antivirals (e.g., nelfinavir), antimalarials (e.g., chloroquine), anesthetics (e.g., halothane), antiarrhythmics (e.g., quinidine), antidepressants (e.g., amitriptyline), antipsychotics (e.g., risperidone), antihistamines (e.g., terfenadine), and cisapride.[65] It is important to be aware of this list because the antimuscarinic effects are additive.

M1 is found in exocrine glands, such as the salivary glands, and in the central nervous system (CNS). The side effect of dry mouth is thought to be due, at least in part, to the inhibitory effect of M1 on the salivary gland. M3 receptors are also known to be important in the salivary gland. Cognitive impairment is another side effect of M1 receptor blockade. In one study of cognitive function, oxybutynin 20 mg caused a temporary effect equivalent to 10–20 years of cognitive decline.[66] The M4 receptor and M5 receptors are believed to be within the CNS, but their function is unknown.

## Efficacy

Despite the theoretical differences among the different AMAs, it is generally agreed that all have similar efficacy.

However, evaluating the overall efficacy of AMAs is diffi-cult because, until very recently, there have been no valid outcome measures for urgency, the key symptom of OAB. The primary efficacy outcome measures for virtually all U.S. Food and Drug Administration (FDA) registration studies were either the change in urge urinary inconti-nence episodes or the change in number of voids per 24 hours.

With those caveats, the results of multiple studies on all anti-muscarinics show a mean decrease in voids per 24 hours of 17%–22%, compared to 8%–15% for that of placebo. Thus, a patient who voided 11 times per day would be expected to void nine times with the AMA versus ten with the placebo. Urge incontinence episodes fell 57%–77%, compared to 33%–58% for placebo. A patient who had two urge incon-tinent episodes a day would be expected to have less than one episode per day with the AMA, and about 1.5 with the placebo.

Despite these results, most patients do not remain on AMA treatment for very long, either because of side effects or lack of efficacy. In one large study of women with OAB who were treated with AMAs and followed for at least 6 months, 6% reported cure and 48% significant improvement, but only 18% were still taking the AMA at 6 months. Side effects caused 40% to stop treatment even though half of these patients thought the drug effective.[67]

### Side Effects
The common side effects of antimuscarinics are mostly due to their effect on muscarinic receptors in the salivary

gland (dry mouth), intestine (constipation), brain (cognitive dysfunction), and iris (blurred vision). To some degree, all antimuscarinics can cause these side effects, but the relative incidences are different.[63] There are two theoretic factors that contribute to the occurrence of side effects: the serum concentration of the active drug or metabolite at the end organ, and the degree of receptor specificity of the AMA.

Serum concentration is dependent upon the dose, route of administration and, for CNS side effects, the degree to which the active drug crosses the blood–brain barrier. Oxybutynin, tolterodine, and fesoterodine are the least specific of the available antimuscarinics. With oral antimuscarinics, increasing dose correlates with increased likelihood of side effects. However, because of unique absorptive properties, side effects of patch and gel preparations do not necessarily increase with increasing dose. In addition to dose, other factors, such as drug metabolites and enzymatic breakdown pathways, also contribute to the genesis of side effects.

### Dry Mouth (Xerostomia)

The most common side effect of AMA is dry mouth (10%–31%), which often causes patients to increase their fluid intake and exacerbate OAB symptoms. Xerostomia can also cause dental cavities, and difficulties with speech (phonation) and eating. The effects of metabolites on the muscarinic receptor affect the incidence of xerostomia. For example, N-deseloxybutynin (DEO) is the primary metabolite of oxybutynin. Oral oxybutynin is metabolized in the liver by the cytochrome P450 system using CYP3a4, and is converted into DEO, which has a higher affinity for the parotid gland and is the main causes of dry mouth in patients taking oxybutynin. The transdermal and gel formulations have a lower incidence of dry mouth because of a smaller amount of CYP3a4 in the skin and, consequently, a smaller amount of conversion to DEO. Oxybutynin ER has a lower incidence of dry mouth because, unlike oxybutynin IR, it is absorbed primarily in the large colon, which has a lower concentration of CYP3a4, rather than in the small bowel. The somewhat lower incidence of xerostomia with fesoterodine and tolterodine are likely because its bioactive agent, 5-hydroxymethyl tolterodine (5-HMT), has less effect on the salivary ducts.[68,69]

### Constipation

Constipation is the second most common reported side effect of AMAs (2%–14%). Because of the presence of the M3 receptor on bowel wall mucosa, all AMAs can cause constipation.[68] However, selective M3 agents tend to have a higher incidence of constipation compared with nonselective agents. Constipation can often be mitigated by laxatives and stool softeners.

### Central Nervous System Side Effects

Central nervous system side effects (impaired memory and cognition, dizziness, somnolence, and insomnia) are thought to be caused by interactions with the M1, M4, and/or M5 receptors. However, for these side effects to occur, the medication needs to cross the blood–brain barrier (the interface between capillary walls and brain substance). Factors that promote diffusion across the blood–brain barrier include drug factors (serum concentration, protein binding, lipid solubility, polarity, and molecular weight) and patient factors. Patient factors that cause breakdown of the blood–brain barrier include altered cerebral blood flow, increased metabolic requirements of brain function, and disease states such as cerebrovascular disease, multiple sclerosis, spinal cord injury, diabetes mellitus, fever, and aging.[68] Oxybutynin is both lipophilic and nonselective and has well-documented CNS effects. In fact, cognitive impairment from M1 receptor blockade with oxybutynin 20 mg was equivalent to 10–20 years of general cognitive decline which was reversible with withdrawal of the medication in one study.[66] Trospium is hydrophilic (not lipophilic) and has a lower incidence of CNS effects.[68] Additionally, M3 receptor-specific medications, such as darifenacin and solifenacin, have demonstrated fewer CNS side effects than oxybutynin.[70]

### Other Side Effects
Other reported side effects include blurry vision (oxybutynin solifenacin, tolterodine), erythema (higher with oxybutynin 5 mg t.i.d.) fatigue (tolterodine 4 mg/d), pruritus (oxybutynin 5 mg t.i.d.), increased sweating (solifenacin 5 mg/d), and an increased risk of urinary retention (oxybutynin 7.5–10 mg t.i.d.) (Table 7).[68]

### Oxybutynin Immediate Release (Ditropan)
Oxybutynin is a nonselective AMA that has been used to treat OAB for over 30 years. It is well absorbed from the

Table 7  Antimuscarinic Agents

| Medi-cation | Dose | Receptor Affinity[89] | Meta-bolism | Side Effects | | |
|---|---|---|---|---|---|---|
| | | | | Dry mouth | Consti-pation | CNS |
| Oxybutynin IR | 5 mg t.i.d. | M1–4 | Hepatic | *** | *** | *** |
| Oxybutynin ER | 4 mg q.d. | M1–4 | Hepatic | ** | ** | ** |
| Oxybutynin patch | 3.9 mg BIW | M1–4 | Hepatic, second-pass | ** | * | ** |
| Oxybutynin gel | 1 gm q.d. | M1–4 | Hepatic, second-pass | ** | * | ** |
| Tolterodine LA | 4 mg q.d. | M1, M2, M3, M5 | Hepatic | *** | ** | * |
| Darifenacin | 7.5/15 mg q.d. | M3 | Hepatic | *** | * ** | * |
| Solifenacin | 5/10 mg q.d. | M3 | Hepatic | ** | * * | * |
| Trospium | 20 mg b.i.d. | M1–5 | Renal | *** | ** | * |
| Fesoterodine | 4/8 mg q.d. | M1, M2, M3, M5 | Hepatic | *** | ** | * |
| * denotes least severe, ** somewhat severe, *** most severe | | | | | | |

gastrointestinal tract and can be taken with or without food. It has a ten-fold greater selectivity for M3 over M2.[71] A short half-life necessitates thrice daily dosing (usually at 5 mg). Contraindications include patients with urinary retention, severely decreased gastric motility, and certain cases of narrow-angle glaucoma.[72] Because oxybutynin is very lipophilic and has a relatively low molecular weight, it easily crosses the blood–brain barrier and has a high risk of CNS side effects. Metabolism occurs through the hepatic CYP3a4 system, and caution is advised for patients taking CYP3a4 inhibitors, such as itraconazole, which can increase serum concentrations and prolong the side effects of oxybutynin. The primary metabolite, DEO, is also bioactive but with higher affinity for the parotid gland M1 and M3 receptor, resulting in xerostomia. Because of the relatively higher incidence of dose-dependent side effects, gradual dose titration is recommended.[73] The necessity of frequent dosing and the relatively higher incidence of side effects make long-term compliance poor, particularly in the elderly.

Because of its short half-life and rapid absorption (time to maximum serum concentration is 0.5–1 hour), oxybutynin IR may be preferable to other, longer-acting, AMAs as an as-needed drug, and it can be given as a single dose in the evening to patients who have nocturia.

### Oxybutynin Extended Release (Ditropan ER)

A long-acting formulation of oxybutynin, oxybutynin ER uses an osmotic system to gradually deliver medicine over a 24-hour period. It can be taken with or without food, and is primarily absorbed in the colon. Peak concentration occurs in 11–13 hours.[74] Because of a lower concentration of CYP3a4 in the colon, there is less DEO production than with the IR formulation, which is one reason for a lower side-effect profile[75] and better tolerability.[76] Oxybutynin ER has a wide dosing range, from 5 to 30 mg, permitting more gradual titration between side effects and benefits.

## Oxybutynin Transdermal Delivery System (Oxytrol TDS)

Because of the absorption and pharmacokinetics of the oxybutynin TDS, steady-state concentrations last as long as 96 hours, permitting twice weekly dosing of the 3.9 mg/d skin patch. For patients who are switched to the TDS from oral oxybutynin preparations, there is no consistent conversion factor.[72] Only small amounts of CYP3a4 are found in skin, and Oxytrol TDS does not undergo first-pass metabolism in the liver, thus resulting in a lower concentration of DEO and a decreased risk of xerostomia.[77]

Application site pruritus (10%–16%) and dermatitis[78] is a unique complication of the TDS and results in discontinuation in about 10% of patients.[79] Antihistamines and topical corticosteroids may be used to mitigate skin reactions.[63]

## Oxybutynin Gel (Gelnique)

Gelnique contains 100 mg of oxybutynin and is applied daily. The gel is quick drying and purportedly minimizes the local irritation seen with TDS. Because it is still absorbed cutaneously, it retains the TDS's favorable side-effect profile. Patients are advised not to shower, bathe, or exercise for at least 1 hour after the application. The most common side effects are local skin reactions and dry mouth, although the incidence of dry mouth is less than with oxybutynin IR tablets.

## Tolterodine Tartrate Immediate and Extended Release (Detrol and Detrol LA)

Tolterodine is a nonspecific AMA acting on both M2 and M3 receptors, usually prescribed as a 4 mg daily tablet. It can be taken with or without food. Initially formulated as an IR tablet, the ER formulation gained popularity after being shown to provide greater symptomatic relief with less dry mouth and generally fewer side effects.[80] Because tolterodine has relatively low lipid solubility, CNS side effects are fewer than those associated oxybutynin.[73] Tolterodine's active metabolite is 5-HMT. Since the conversion is catalyzed by an enzyme found in the liver, 5-HMT serum levels are erratic in patients with liver dysfunction, and in these patients, the drug should be used with caution.

## Darifenacin Hydrobromide (Enablex)

Darifenacin was formulated as the first M3-receptor–specific AMA, and is dosed at 7.5 mg and 15 mg daily. It is well absorbed and can be taken with or without food without altering its bioavailability. It is also processed by the liver and should be used with caution in patients with hepatic impairment. Because of M3 specificity, darifenacin has been demonstrated to have lower CNS side effects than oxybutynin, and had equivalent memory effects to a placebo. Due to its M3 affinity, it has higher rates of constipation than the nonselective AMAs.[63]

## Solifenacin Succinate (Vesicare)

Solifenacin, like darifenacin, is a single daily dose M3-specific AMA that is dosed in 5 or 10 mg tablets that can be taken with or without food. Peak plasma levels (tmax) occur between 3–8 hours after oral ingestion, therefore taking the medication prior to bedtime may not help with nocturia symptoms. It is metabolized by the CYP3a4 cytochrome P450 system, and caution is advised when giving this to patients with hepatic impairment.[81] Because it is hydrophilic and M3 specific, CNS side effects are less severe than with oxybutynin.

### Fesoterodine Fumarate (Toviaz)

Fesoterodine is administered as a 4 or 8 mg daily dose that can be taken with or without food. The parent compound, fesoterodine, has minimal antimuscarinic activity and is rapidly metabolized to 5-HMT, a nonspecific AMA.[82] Pharmokinetic variability is low among different patients.[83] 5-HMT is further metabolized in the liver by the cytochrome P450 system into minimally active metabolites. Although both tolterodine and fesoterodine are metabolized into 5-HMT, the conversion of tolterodine occurs through the CYP3a4 system, which has much greater variability in expression and effect. Fesoterodine is an ideal medication for those patients for whom there is concern about excretion and impairment of hepatic function.[84]

### Trospium Chloride (Sanctura)

Trospium is a nonselective antimuscarinic, but CNS effects are low because it is not lipophilic. It was initially formulated as a twice-daily 20 mg tablet; later an ER formulation was added. Food reduces its bioavailability, so it should be taken on an empty stomach. It is the only antimuscarinic not processed by the cytochrome P450 system, and it is cleared completely by the kidneys. The dose should be decreased to 20 mg daily for those with a low creatinine clearance. Because of the lack of hepatic metabolism, it may have comparatively fewer interactions with other medications, making it a good first option for the elderly or those taking multiple medications.[63] Furthermore, as a selective M3 agent, it has a lower incidence of dry mouth than oxybutynin.[85]

### Non-Antimuscarinic Medications

Non-muscarinic agents, which are not approved for OAB, include tricyclic antidepressants (TCAs), and other antispasmodics/analgesics such as flavoxate.[86, 87]

### Conclusions About Pharmacologic Treatment

- All antimuscarinics have similar efficacy.
- All antimuscarinics have a similar side-effect profile, but the incidence of individual side effects may vary based on route of administration, receptor specificity, chemical structure, and metabolic breakdown pathways.
- Generally, controlled-release medications have less adverse events.
- Long-term compliance for all of the antimuscarinics is low.[88]
- In elderly patients or others in whom there is concern about cognitive function, a selective M3 receptor blocker or one that does not have an affinity for crossing the blood–brain barrier is advisable.
- For those who have preexisting constipation, nonselective antimuscarinics are preferable to M3 selective blockers due to the presence of M3 receptors in the bowel.

- In patients with hepatic impairment, trospium or fesoterodine may be preferable because they are not processed by the CYP3a4 system. Darifenacin should be avoided in patients with severe hepatic impairment.

## Pelvic Floor Muscle Training and Biofeedback

Pelvic floor muscle training (PFMT) and biofeedback have been used for decades to treat OAB. Pelvic floor muscle training is analogous to a coach and an athlete, wherein the patient is taught how to use and condition her pelvic floor muscles. Biofeedback and other devices, such as vaginal cones, and electrical stimulation are adjunctive techniques.[90] It has been proposed that contraction of the pelvic floor, through an unknown neurologic reflex, shuts off the involuntary detrusor contraction that causes urgency in some patients.[91–93] Pelvic floor muscle training can be conducted by the patient herself after proper instruction from a therapist, with or without biofeedback, and through the use of weighted vaginal cones.[90] Several studies have shown no advantage to biofeedback over supervised exercises,[90,94] but biofeedback may be useful in patients who do not understand how to contract their muscles.

Biofeedback involves monitoring body functions and conveying the information in real-time, with the goal of teaching the patient to recognize and control these functions.[95] Biofeedback for OAB has two applications: to teach the patient how to control the pelvic floor muscles, and to strengthen those muscles. We believe that biofeedback is most effective when combined with behavior modification.[59] The patient is taught how to contract the pelvic floor and to do so whenever an uncomfortable urge to void is felt. By contracting the sphincter, incontinence is prevented during the involuntary bladder contraction, and, in addition, this activates the neurologic reflex alluded to earlier that shuts off the bladder contraction, thus enabling the patient to comfortably find a bathroom.

Biofeedback technique utilizes either a pressure or EMG sensor placed in the vagina, perineum, or rectum. The patient is taught how to contract, and the strength and duration of each muscle contraction is displayed on a screen or signaled by a buzzing sound. The sessions are usually scheduled once a week, or the patient may purchase or rent a unit for home use. Based on the progress made each week, an exercise program is planned for the following week. The long-term efficacy of biofeedback has not been determined in well-designed studies, but there have not been any reported complications. Short-term studies with 6-week to 6-month follow-up have suggested between 54% and 87% improvement in incontinence.[96,97] One meta-analysis found biofeedback with pelvic floor exercises to be superior to pelvic floor exercises alone.[98]

### Electrical Stimulation

Electrical stimulation of the pelvic floor has been advocated by some for OAB. It is hypothesized that repetitive stimulation results in increased strength and tone, and also, through a negative feedback system, inhibits detrusor contraction. It is performed by placing a stimulation electrode either in or near the vagina, rectum, perineum,[99] or at the posterior tibial nerve at the ankle.[100] The electrode may be a surface patch, or it may be shaped like a balloon (for the vagina) or an hourglass (for the rectum). The stimulation sessions are usually scheduled at weekly or biweekly intervals.

### Absorbent Pads and Other Forms of Protection

Many kinds of absorbent pads, panty liners, and adult diapers are available for both men and women. For patients with small amounts of urine loss, panty liners or absorbant pads may be sufficient; for more urine loss, diapers are necessary. Other issues to consider are the absorbancy of the diapers, the size and presence of adjustable straps, and the presence of a wicking system to keep skin dry. A complete list of current products is available in many catalogues. The most user-friendly and extensive catalogue is the one published by The National Association for Continence, which can be contacted on its website (www.nafc.org).

## SURGICAL TREATMENT

Surgical treatment of OAB is considered under two circumstances: when there is an underlying remediable condition (Table 3), and when the OAB symptoms have proven refractory to nonsurgical treatments. For refractory OAB unassociated with a remedial condition, Botox injections, neuromodulation, enterocystoplasty, and urinary diversion may be considered.

### Botox (Botulinum Toxin)

Botox injections (not approved by the FDA for OAB treatment) into the detrusor muscle have recently shown positive effects in treating patients with refractory neurogenic DO, and this treatment also shows promise in patients with non-neurogenic etiologies.[101–104]

Seven different serotypes of the clostridial botulinum neurotoxin (A–G) are available, but at present only Botox A and B have been used to treat OAB. The primary mode of action is thought to be inhibition of detrusor contractions through inhibition of acetylcholine and adenosine triphosphate (ATP). In addition, there is some evidence that Botox A may have sensory and antinociceptive effects.

## Neuromodulation

Neuromodulation refers to an implantable electrical stimulation device that has been shown to be effective in some patients with refractory OAB. The system is comprised of two parts: an electrical lead that is placed near the third sacral nerve and an implantable neurostimulator. The device is implanted in two stages: a percutaneous test stimulation to determine whether the treatment is likely to be effective and the implant procedure. Both are done in the outpatient setting with local anesthesia and sedation. In the first session, the lead is passed through the third sacral foramen and the wires are brought out through the skin and connected to the neurostimulator. The patient uses the device for 2–4 weeks and, if it is effective, the permanent implant is performed; if not, the leads are removed. Once the device is implanted, subsequent magnetic resonance imaging (MRI) studies are contraindicated.

In most studies of neuromodulation, the primary outcome measure has been a >50% reduction in OAB symptoms at 6 months and, using that metric, the success rate has ranged from 56% to 90%.[105,106] Complications are minor and include pain, lead migration, technical problems, decreased efficacy, and infection.[108]

### Augmentation Enterocystoplasty, Ileovesicostomy, and Urinary Diversion

These operations are generally considered only as a last resort when the patient deems the symptoms bad enough to warrant a major abdominal operation. In augmentation enterocystoplasty, part of the intestine (the ileum or ileocecal segment) is detached from the rest of the bowel, reconfigured, and anastomosed to the bladder. The purpose of the operation is to greatly increase bladder capacity and to prevent DO. The success rate is in excess of 90%, and afterward the patient may void naturally or may require intermittent self-catheterization.[109–111]

For patients with disabilities that make catheterizing through the urethra impractical, a continent abdominal stoma may be created for intermittent catheterization, or an ileovesicostomy or ileal loop may be considered. The complications are the same as for any other major abdominal operation, including wound infection, which is particularly common in obese patients and those with neurologic bladder. There are reports of troublesome diarrhea and malabsorption of vitamin $B_{12}$ requiring supplements. Over the long-term there is a risk of urinary tract infection, urolithiasis, and renal failure, but all of these risks are much less than that of other treatments for refractory OAB—indwelling catheters and supravesical urinary diversion.

For patients in whom intermittent catheterization is impractical, a urinary conduit will relieve the OAB symptoms, but at the cost of a higher rate of infection, urolithiasis, and renal failure.

## INCONTINENCE-ASSOCIATED DERMATITIS (DIAPER RASH)

### Causes

Incontinence-associated dermatitis, or diaper rash, occurs in 5.6%–50% of adults with incontinence.[112] For patients with OAB-causing incontinence (urge incontinence) or for those who have OAB combined with stress incontinence (mixed incontinence), prevention and management is critical to improving quality of life and potentially preventing life-threatening infections.

Risk factors for dermatitis secondary to urinary incontinence include exogenous and endogenous factors. Exogenous factors include the length of time and amount of exposure to urine. The urine itself creates a warm, moist environment that enhances the growth of microorganisms and enhances irritation from heat and sweating. Other exogenous factors that affect the development of a rash are the presence of fecal incontinence, type of diaper used, and frequency of diaper changes. Infrequent diaper changes will increase the time and volume of urine exposure to the skin.

Endogenous factors include the patient's age, gender, and immune status, and the presence of other skin diseases. The stratum corneum, the outer layer of the epidermis, provides a critical barrier to microorganisms. When skin is exposed to moisture, permeability increases and the barrier function decreases. The composition of this layer changes with age, and this makes the skin of older patients more susceptible to maceration and dermatitis when soaked with urine. Furthermore, older patients who develop incontinence-associated dermatitis are at an increased risk of developing a secondary infection.

Women with incontinence have a higher incidence of incontinence-associated dermatitis. Although the reason for this is unclear, it may be hormonal differences or simply that, in women, a greater amount of leaked urine is exposed to the skin prior to being absorbed by the diaper.[113]

The presence of previous skin diseases may decrease the body's natural resistance and increase the likelihood of maceration. In the elderly, diaper rash may also mask underlying skin conditions. In one prospective study of 46 patients with adult incontinence-associated dermatitis, 63% had candidiasis, 16% irritant dermatitis, 11% eczema, and 11% psoriasis.[114]

### Treatment

Skin moistened by urine has increased skin pH, which increases bacterial colonization. Urine in contact with the skin leads to maceration of the skin which, in turn, encourages infiltration by *Candida* or bacteria. Ideally, treatment for incontinence-associated dermatitis includes permanently correcting the incontinence. Because this is not always possible, supportive treatment should include minimizing the time and amount of urine that is in contact with the skin.

The use of a skin care protocol decreases the risk of dermatitis and secondary infection. This protocol may include a fixed plan for frequency of pad or diaper changes, the amount of barrier used, routine examinations to diagnose early dermatitis, and periodic cleaning. Gentle skin cleansers may decrease the pathogenic bacterial load. Hypoallergenic diapers or pads with minimally irritating fasteners should be used and changed frequently. The addition of Diflucan or antifungal creams is useful because patients may also have a concomitant candidal infection. In one study of patients who developed a secondary candidal infection, antifungal agents cured 32% of patients, improved 56%, and left only 12% unchanged or worsened.[114] Because of compromised skin integrity, secondary bacterial infections can also occur and should be aggressively treated with appropriate oral antibiotics. When bacterial infection is suspected, it is important to culture the skin before treating with oral antibiotics, given the growing incidence of resistant *Staphylococcus aureus*, vancomycin-resistant enterococcus, and other gram-negative organisms that can be isolated.

In addition to frequent diaper changes and appropriate antimicrobial therapy, skin barriers may be useful. It is helpful to use a product that replicates skin pH as closely as possible. Products that provide a barrier function include zinc oxide, which can be combined with an antiseptic formulation. Skin moisturizers such as petroleum jelly also provide a barrier between the skin and the diaper to decrease the incidence of dermatitis.[115]

## APPENDIX A

Overactive Bladder Symptom Score:

### OAB and Incontinence Questionnaire

NAME: _____DATE: _____

**Instructions: Please mark only one answer for each question and do not handwrite any answers.** Most symptoms vary from day to day. We understand that if you check off more than one, you feel that you will be providing more information about your condition. Please do not do this. Just check the box that best describes you. You will have the opportunity to discuss your symptoms in more detail with your doctor.

### 1. How often do you usually urinate during the day?

____ No more often than once in 4 hours

____ About every 3–4 hours

____ About every 2–3 hours

____ About every 1–2 hours

____ At least once an hour

### 2. How many times do you usually urinate at night (from the time you go to bed until the time you wake up for the day)?

____ 0–1 times

____ 2 times

____ 3 times

____ 4 times

____ 5 or more times

### 3. What is the reason that you usually urinate?

\_\_\_\_ Out of convenience (no urge or desire)

\_\_\_\_ Because I have a mild urge or desire (but can delay urination for over an hour if I have to)

\_\_\_\_ Because I have a moderate urge or desire (but can delay urination for more than 10 but less than 60 minutes if I have to)

\_\_\_\_ Because I have a severe urge or desire (but can delay urination for less than 10 minutes if I have to)

\_\_\_\_ Because I have desperate urge or desire (must stop what I am doing and go immediately)

### 4. Once you get the urge or desire to urinate, how long can you usually postpone it comfortably?

\_\_\_\_ More than 60 minutes

\_\_\_\_ About 30–60 minutes

\_\_\_\_ About 10–30 minutes

\_\_\_\_ A few minutes (less than 10 minutes)

\_\_\_\_ Must go immediately

### 5. How often do you get a sudden urge or desire to urinate that makes you want to stop what you are doing and rush to the bathroom?

\_\_\_\_ Never

\_\_\_\_ Rarely

\_\_\_\_ A few times a month

\_\_\_\_ A few times a week

\_\_\_\_ At least once a day

6. How often do you get a sudden urge or desire to urinate that makes you want to stop what you are doing and rush to the bathroom but you don't get there in time (i.e., you leak urine or wet pads)?

\_\_\_\_ Never

\_\_\_\_ Rarely

\_\_\_\_ A few times a month

\_\_\_\_ A few times a week

\_\_\_\_ At least once a day

7. In your opinion, how good is your bladder control?

\_\_\_\_ Perfect control

\_\_\_\_ Very good

\_\_\_\_ Good

\_\_\_\_ Poor

\_\_\_\_ No control at all

## APPENDIX B

Overactive Bladder Diary

Name: _____ Date: _____

Time of day diary started: _____ ☐ AM ☐ PM

Time you went to bed _____
Time you got up for the day _____

| Time of urination and /or incontinence episode | Why did you urinate at this time? (See question (a) for responses) | Amount of urination (measure with a cup in cc's, mL's or ounces) | Incontinence grade (See question (b) below for responses) |
|---|---|---|---|
| 1 | | | |
| 2 | | | |
| 3 | | | |
| 4 | | | |
| 5 | | | |
| 6 | | | |
| 7 | | | |
| 8 | | | |
| 9 | | | |
| 10 | | | |
| 11 | | | |
| 12 | | | |
| 13 | | | |
| 14 | | | |
| 15 | | | |

Please select the number next to your answer and use it for your response to the above questions.

**(a)** Why did you urinate?  **(b)** Incontinence grade.

**(0)** Out of convenience (no urge or desire)  **(0)** Grade 1 – Some drops

**(1)** Because I have a mild (but can delay urination for over urge an hour if I have to)  **(1)** Grade 2 – Moderate loss (wet underpants)

**(2)** Grade 3 – Extensive loss (wet outer clothes)  **(2)** Because I have a moderate urge (but can delay urination for more than 10 but less than 60 minutes if I have to)

**(3)** Because I have a severe urge (but can delay urination for less than 10 minutes)

**(4)** Because I have desperate urge (must stop what I am doing and go immediately)

OFFICE USE

**Total 24-hour output** _____  **# of voids** _____
**MVV =** _____

**Day volume** _____  **# voids**
**Night volume** _____  **# voids** _____  **NPI** _____

## REFERENCES

1. Milsom, I., et al. How widespread are the symptoms of an overactive bladder and how are they managed? A population-based prevalence study. *BJU Int* 2001;87(9):760–6.

2. Stewart, W., et al. The prevalence and impact of overactive bladder in the U.S: results from the NOBLE program. *Neurorol Urodynam* 2001;20(406):8.

3. Abrams, P., et al. The standardisation of terminology of lower urinary tract function: report from the Standardisation Sub-committee of the International Continence Society. *Neurourol Urodynam* 2002;21(2):167–78.

4. Blaivas, J.G., et al. Two types of urgency. *Neurourol Urodynam* 2009;28(3):188–90.

5. Fusco, F., et al. Videourodynamic studies in men with lower urinary tract symptoms: a comparison of community based versus referral urological practices. *J Urol* 2001;166(3): 910–3.

6. Sriplakich, S., & Promwatcharanon, K. The resolution of detrusor over activity after medical and surgical treatment in patients with bladder outlet obstruction. *J Med Assoc Thai* 2007;90(11): 2326–31.

7. Kageyama, S., et al. Can persisting detrusor hyperreflexia be predicted after transurethral prostatectomy for benign prostatic hypertrophy? *Neurourol Urodynam* 2000;19(3):233–40.

8. Blaivas, J.G., Groutz, A., & Verhaaren, M. Does the method of cystometry affect the incidence of involuntary detrusor contractions? A prospective randomized urodynamic study. *Neurourol Urodynam* 2001;20(2):141–5.

9. Flisser, A.J., Walmsley, K., & Blaivas, J.G. Urodynamic classification of patients with symptoms of overactive bladder. *J Urol* 2003;169(2):529–33; discussion 533–4.

10. Fitzgerald, M.P., Brubaker, L. Variability of 24-hour voiding diary variables among asymptomatic women. *J Urol* 2003;169(1):207–9.

11. Fitzgerald, M.P., Stablein, U., & Brubaker, L. Urinary habits among asymptomatic women. *Am J Obstet Gynecol* 2002; 187(5):1384–8.

12. Parsons, M., et al. Bladder diary patterns in detrusor overactivity and urodynamic stress incontinence. *Neurourol Urodynam* 2007;26(6):800–6.

13. Bing, M.H., et al. Prevalence and bother of nocturia, and causes of sleep interruption in a Danish population of men and women aged 60–80 years. *BJU Int* 2006;98(3): 599–604.

14. Coyne, K.S., et al. The prevalence of nocturia and its effect on health-related quality of life and sleep in a community sample in the USA. *BJU Int* 2003;92(9):948–54.

15. Yoshimura, K., et al. Prevalence of and risk factors for nocturia: analysis of a health screening program. *Int J Urol* 2004; 11(5):282–7.

16. Barker, J.C., & Mitteness, L.S. Nocturia in the elderly. *Gerontologist* 1988;28(1):99–104.

17. Gourova, L.W., et al. Predictive factors for nocturia in elderly men: a cross-sectional study in 21 general practices. *BJU Int* 2006;97(3):528–32.

18. Blaivas, J.G., et al. The urgency perception score: validation and test-retest. *J Urol* 2007;177(1):199–202.

19. Nixon, A., et al. A validated patient reported measure of urinary urgency severity in overactive bladder for use in clinical trials. *J Urol* 2005;174(2):604–7.

20. Zinner, N., et al. The overactive bladder-symptom composite score: a composite symptom score of toilet voids, urgency severity and urge urinary incontinence in patients with overactive bladder. *J Urol* 2005;173(5):1639–43.

21. Marks, B.K., et al. Differential diagnosis of overactive bladder in men. *J Urol* 2009;182(6):2814–7.

22. Dmochowski, R.R., & Staskin, D. Overactive bladder in men: special considerations for evaluation and management. *Urology* 2002;60(5 Suppl 1):56–62; discussion 62–3.

23. Hyman, M.J., Groutz, A, & Blaivas, J.G. Detrusor instability in men: correlation of lower urinary tract symptoms with urodynamic findings. *J Urol* 2001;166(2):550–2; discussion 553.

24. Kaplan, S.A., et al. Differential diagnosis of prostatism: a 12-year retrospective analysis of symptoms, urodynamics and satisfaction with therapy. *J Urol* 1996;155(4):1305–8.

25. Blaivas, J.G. The neurophysiology of micturition: a clinical study of 550 patients. *J Urol* 1982;127(5):958–63.

26. Hebjorn, S., et al. Detrusor hyperreflexia. A survey on its etiology and treatment. *Scand J Urol Nephrol* 1976;10(2):103–9.

27. Kolominsky-Rabas, P.L., et al. Impact of urinary incontinence after stroke: results from a prospective population-based stroke register. *Neurourol Urodynam* 2003;22(4):322–7.

28. Chou, E.C., et al. Effective treatment for mixed urinary incontinence with a pubovaginal sling. *J Urol* 2003;170(2 Pt 1):494–7.

29. Griffiths, D.J., et al. Relationship of fluid intake to voluntary micturition and urinary incontinence in geriatric patients. *Neurourol Urodynam* 1993;12(1):1–7.

30. Groutz, A., et al. Noninvasive outcome measures of urinary incontinence and lower urinary tract symptoms: a multicenter study of micturition diary and pad tests. *J Urol* 2000;164(3 Pt 1):698–701.

31. Yoon, E., & Swift, S. A comparison of maximum cystometric bladder capacity with maximum environmental voided volumes. *Int Urogynecol J Pelvic Floor Dysfunct* 1998;9(2):78–82.

32. Diokno, A.C., Wells, T.J., & Brink, C.A. Comparison of self-reported voided volume with cystometric bladder capacity. *J Urol* 1987;137(4):698–700.

33. Asplund, R. The nocturnal polyuria syndrome (NPS). *Gen Pharmacol* 1995;26(6):1203–9.

34. Weiss, J.P., et al. Nocturia in adults: etiology and classification. *Neurourol Urodynam* 1998;17(5):467–72.

35. Weiss, J.P., et al. Evaluation of the etiology of nocturia in men: the nocturia and nocturnal bladder capacity indices. *Neurourol Urodynam* 1999;18(6):559–65.

36. van Dijk, L., Kooij, D.G., & Schellevis, F.G. Nocturia in the Dutch adult population. *BJU Int* 2002;90(7):644–8.

37. Weiss, J.P., et al. Age related pathogenesis of nocturia in patients with overactive bladder. *J Urol* 2007;178(2):548–51.

38. Kirkland, J.L., et al. Patterns of urine flow and electrolyte excretion in healthy elderly people. *Br Med J (Clin Res Ed)* 1983;287(6406):1665–7.

39. Matthiesen, T.B., et al. Nocturnal polyuria and natriuresis in male patients with nocturia and lower urinary tract symptoms. *J Urol* 1996;156(4):1292–9.

40. Asplund, R., et al. Nocturia, depression and antidepressant medication. *BJU Int* 2005;95(6):820–3.

41. Endeshaw, Y.W., et al. Sleep-disordered breathing and nocturia in older adults. *J Am Geriatr Soc* 2004;52(6):957–60.

42. Fitzgerald, M.P., et al. The association of nocturia with cardiac disease, diabetes, body mass index, age and diuretic use: results from the BACH survey. *J Urol* 2007;177(4):1385–9.

43. Fitzgerald, M.P., Mulligan, M., & Parthasarathy, S. Nocturic frequency is related to severity of obstructive sleep apnea, improves with continuous positive airways treatment. *Am J Obstet Gynecol* 2006;194(5): 399–403.

44. Graugaard-Jensen, C., Rittig, S., & Djurhuus, J.C. Nocturia and circadian blood pressure profile in healthy elderly male volunteers. *J Urol* 2006;176(3):1034–9; discussion 1039.

45. Partinen, M. Epidemiology of obstructive sleep apnea syndrome. *Curr Opin Pulm Med* 1995;1(6):482–7.

46. Rembratt, A., & Weiss, J. Pathogenesis of nocturia in the elderly: relationship of functional bladder capacity to nocturnal urine output. *J Urol* 2001;165 (Suppl):250.

47. Van Cauter, E., & Copinschi, G. Altered hormonal secretions in aging: roles of sleep and circadian rhythms. First Congress on the Aging Male, Geneva, 1998.

48. Wall, L.L., DeLancey, J.O.L., & Norton, P.A., eds. *Practical urogynecology.* Baltimore: Williams & Wilkins, 1993; 293–315.

49. Blaivas, J.G., et al. Validation of the overactive bladder symptom score. *J Urol* 2007;178(2):543–7; discussion 547.

50. De Wachter, S., & Wyndaele, J.J. Frequency-volume charts: a tool to evaluate bladder sensation. *Neurourol Urodynam* 2003;22(7):638–42.

51. Larsson, G., & Victor, A. Micturition patterns in a healthy female population, studied with a frequency/volume chart. *Scand J Urol Nephrol Suppl* 1988;114:53–7.

52. Lose, G., Gammelgaard, J., & Jorgensen, T. The one-hour pad-weighing test: reproducibility and the correlation between the test result, start volume in the bladder and the diuresis. *Neurourol Urodynam* 1986;5(17).

53. O'Sullivan, R., et al. Definition of mild, moderate and severe incontinence on the 24-hour pad test. *BJOG* 2004;111(8):859–62.

54. Bump, R.C., et al. The standardization of terminology of female pelvic organ prolapse and pelvic floor dysfunction. *Am J Obstet Gynecol* 1996;175(1):10–7.

55. Blaivas, J.G., Zayed, A.A., & Labib, K.B. The bulbocaverno-sus reflex in urology: a prospective study of 299 patients. *J Urol* 1981;126(2):197–9.

56. Blaivas, J.G., et al. *Atlas of urodynamics*, 2nd ed. Malden, MA: Blackwell Publishing, 2007; 256.

57. Burgio, K.L., & Goode, P.S. Behavioral interventions for incontinence in ambulatory geriatric patients. *Am J Med Sci* 1997;314(4): 257–61.

58. Burgio, K.L., Locher, J.L., & Goode, P.S. Combined behav-ioral and drug therapy for urge incontinence in older women. *J Am Geriatr Soc* 2000;48(4):370–4.

59. Burgio, K.L. Influence of behavior modification on overactive bladder. *Urology* 2002;60(5 Suppl 1):72–6; discussion 77.

60. Fantl, J.A., et al. Efficacy of bladder training in older women with urinary incontinence. *JAMA* 1991;265(5):609–13.

61. Chapple, C.R., Yamanishi, T., & Chess-Williams, R. Muscarinic receptor subtypes and management of the overactive bladder. *Urology* 2002;60(5 Suppl 1):82–8; discussion 88–9.

62. Yamanishi, T., Chapple, C.R., & Chess-Williams, R. Which muscarinic receptor is important in the bladder? *World J Urol* 2001;19(5):299–306.

63. Chughtai, B., Levin, R., & De, E. Choice of antimuscarinic agents for overactive bladder in the older patient: focus on darifenacin. *Clin Interv Aging* 2008;3(3):503–9.

64. Roden, D.M. Drug-induced prolongation of the QT interval. *N Engl J Med* 2004;350(10):1013–22.

65. Jayasinghe, R., Registrar, S., & Kovoor, P. Drugs and the QTc interval. *Aust Prescr* 2002;25:63–65.

66. Kay, G., et al. Differential effects of the antimuscarinic agents darifenacin and oxybutynin ER on memory in older subjects. *Eur Urol* 2006;50(2):317–26.

67. Kelleher, C.J., et al. A medium-term analysis of the sub-jective efficacy of treatment for women with detrusor

instability and low bladder compliance. *Br J Obstet Gynaecol* 1997;104(9):988–93.

68. Chapple, C., et al. The effects of antimuscarinic treatments in overactive bladder: a systematic review and meta-analysis. *Eur Urol* 2005;48(1):5–26.

69. Sellers, D.J., & McKay, N. Developments in the pharmacotherapy of the overactive bladder. *Curr Opin Urol* 2007;17(4):223–30.

70. Kay, G.G., & Granville, L.J. Antimuscarinic agents: implications and concerns in the management of overactive bladder in the elderly. *Clin Ther* 2005;27(1): 27–38; quiz 139–40.

71. Nilvebrant, L., et al. Tolterodine--a new bladder-selective antimuscarinic agent. *Eur J Pharmacol* 1997;327(2–3):195–207.

72. McCrery, R.J., & Appell, R.A. Oxybutynin: an overview of the available formulations. *Ther Clin Risk Manag* 2006; 2(1):19–24.

73. Yamaguchi, O., et al. Clinical guidelines for overactive bladder. *Int J Urol* 2009;16(2):126–42.

74. Siddiqui, M.A., Perry, C.M., & Scott, L.J. Oxybutynin extended-release: a review of its use in the management of overactive bladder. *Drugs* 2004;64(8):885–912.

75. Arisco, A., Brantly, E., & Kraus, S. Oxybutynin extended release for the management of overactive bladder: a clinical review. *Drug Des Devel Ther* 2009;3:151–61.

76. Anderson, R.U., et al. Once daily controlled versus immediate release oxybutynin chloride for urge urinary incontinence. OROS Oxybutynin Study Group. *J Urol* 1999;161(6):1809–12.

77. Davila, G.W. Transdermal oxybutynin: a new treatment for overactive bladder. *Expert Opin Pharmacother* 2003;4(12): 2315–24.

78. Schaefer, W. Comparison of the efficacy, safety, and tolerability of propiverine and oxybutynin for the treatment of

overactive bladder syndrome. *Int J Urol* 2007;14(7):670; author reply 670–1.

79. Dmochowski, R.R., et al. Comparative efficacy and safety of transdermal oxybutynin and oral tolterodine versus placebo in previously treated patients with urge and mixed urinary incontinence. *Urology* 2003;62(2):237–42.

80. Van Kerrebroeck, P., et al. Tolterodine once-daily: superior efficacy and tolerability in the treatment of the overactive bladder. *Urology* 2001;57(3):414–21.

81. Basra, R.K., et al. A review of adherence to drug therapy in patients with overactive bladder. *BJU Int* 2008;102(7):774–9.

82. Ellsworth, P., Berriman, S.J., & Brodsky, M. Fesoterodine: a new agent for treating overactive bladder. *Am J Manag Care* 2009;15(4 Suppl): S115–7.

83. Wyndaele, J.J., et al. Effects of flexible-dose fesoterodine on overactive bladder symptoms and treatment satisfaction: an open-label study. *Int J Clin Pract* 2009;63(4):560–7.

84. Simon, H.U., & Malhotra, B. The pharmacokinetic profile of fesoterodine: similarities and differences to tolterodine. *Swiss Med Wkly* 2009;139(9–10):146–51.

85. Zinner, N., et al. Trospium chloride improves overactive bladder symptoms: a multicenter phase III trial. *J Urol* 2004;171(6 Pt 1):2311–5, quiz 2435.

86. Milani, R., et al. Comparison of flavoxate hydrochloride in daily dosages of 600 versus 1200 mg for the treatment of urgency and urge incontinence. *J Int Med Res* 1988;16(3):244–8.

87. Chapple, C.R., et al. Double-blind, placebo-controlled, cross-over study of flavoxate in the treatment of idiopathic detrusor instability. *Br J Urol* 1990;66(5):491–4.

88. Kelleher, C.J., et al. Long-term health-related quality of life of patients receiving extended-release tolterodine for overactive bladder. *Am J Manag Care* 2002;8(19 Suppl):S616–30.

89. Hegde, S.S. Muscarinic receptors in the bladder: from basic research to therapeutics. *Br J Pharmacol* 2006;147(Suppl 2): S80–7.

90. Wilson, P.D., et al. Adult conservative management. In P. Abrams, et al., eds., *3rd International Consultation on Incontinence*. Paris: Health Publications Ltd., 2005; 855–964.

91. Godec, C., Cass, A.S., & Ayala, G.F. Bladder inhibition with functional electrical stimulation. *Urology* 1975;6(6):663–6.

92. Morrison, J.F. The excitability of the micturition reflex. *Scand J Urol Nephrol Suppl* 1995;175:21–5.

93. de Groat, W.C., et al. Neural control of the urethra. *Scand J Urol Nephrol Suppl* 2001;207:35–43; discussion 106–25.

94. Burgio, K.L., et al. Behavioral training with and without biofeedback in the treatment of urge incontinence in older women: a randomized controlled trial. *JAMA* 2002;288(18):2293–9.

95. Smith, D.A., & Newman, D.K. Basic elements of biofeedback therapy for pelvic muscle rehabilitation. *Urol Nurs* 1994;14(3):130–5.

96. Susset, J.G., Galea, G., & Read, L. Biofeedback therapy for female incontinence due to low urethral resistance. *J Urol* 1990;143(6):1205–8.

97. Burns, P.A., et al. Treatment of stress incontinence with pelvic floor exercises and biofeedback. *J Am Geriatr Soc* 1990; 38(3):341–4.

98. Weatherall, M. Biofeedback or pelvic floor muscle exercises for female genuine stress incontinence: a meta-analysis of trials identified in a systematic review. *BJU Int* 1999; 83(9):1015–6.

99. Bo, K. Effect of electrical stimulation on stress and urge urinary incontinence. Clinical outcome and practical recommendations based on randomized controlled trials. *Acta Obstet Gynecol Scand Suppl* 1998;168:3–11.

100. Peters, K.M., et al. Randomized trial of percutaneous tibial nerve stimulation versus extended-release tolterodine: results from the overactive bladder innovative therapy trial. *J Urol* 2009;182(3):1055–61.

101. Wefer, B., et al. Treatment outcomes and resource use of patients with neurogenic detrusor overactivity receiving botulinum toxin A (BOTOX(R)) therapy in Germany. *World J Urol*, 2009; August 20 [Epub ahead of print].

102. Karsenty, G., et al. Botulinum toxin A (Botox) intradetrusor injections in adults with neurogenic detrusor overactivity/ neurogenic overactive bladder: a systematic literature review. *Eur Urol* 2008;53(2):275–87.

103. Dmochowski, R., & Sand, P.K. Botulinum toxin A in the overactive bladder: current status and future directions. *BJU Int* 2007;99(2):247–62.

104. Schmid, D.M., et al. Experience with 100 cases treated with botulinum-A toxin injections in the detrusor muscle for idiopathic overactive bladder syndrome refractory to anticholinergics. *J Urol* 2006;176(1):177–85.

105. Chartier-Kastler, E. Sacral neuromodulation for treating the symptoms of overactive bladder syndrome and non-obstructive urinary retention: >10 years of clinical experience. *BJU Int* 2008;101(4):417–23.

106. Campbell, J.D., et al. Treatment success for overactive bladder with urinary urge incontinence refractory to oral antimuscarinics: a review of published evidence. *BMC Urol* 2009;9:18.

107. van Kerrebroeck, P., et al. Desmopressin in the treatment of nocturia: a double-blind, placebo-controlled study. *Eur Urol* 2007;52(1):221–9.

108. Hijaz, A., et al. Complications and troubleshooting of two-stage sacral neuromodulation therapy: a single-institution experience. *Urology* 2006;68(3):533–7.

109. Flood, H.D., et al. Long-term results and complications using augmentation cystoplasty in reconstructive urology. *Neurourol Urodynam* 1995;14(4):297–309.

110. Blaivas, J.G., et al. Long-term followup of augmentation enterocystoplasty and continent diversion in patients with benign disease. *J Urol* 2005;173(5):1631–4.

111. Herschorn, S., & Hewitt, R.J. Patient perspective of long-term outcome of augmentation cystoplasty for neurogenic bladder. *Urology* 1998;52(4):672–8.

112. Gray, M., et al. Incontinence-associated dermatitis: a consensus. *J Wound Ostomy Continence Nurs* 2007;34(1):45–54; quiz 55–56.

113. Slodownik, D., Lee, A., & Nixon, R. Irritant contact dermatitis: a review. *Australia J Dermatol* 2008;49(1):1–9; quiz 10–11.

114. Foureur, N., et al. Prospective aetiological study of diaper dermatitis in the elderly. *Br J Dermatol* 2006;155(5):941–6.

115. Beeckman, D., et al. Prevention and treatment of incontinence-associated dermatitis: literature review. *J Adv Nurs* 2009;65(6):1141–54.